MW00843443

HYPOTHYROIDISM

The Ultimate - Hypothyroidism Solution! Jumpstart Weight Loss With: Natural Remedies, Hypothyroidism Diet, & Clean Eating

2nd EDITION

© Copyright 2015 - All rights reserved.

In no way is it legal to reproduce, duplicate, or transmit any part of this document in either electronic means or in printed format. Recording of this publication is strictly prohibited and any storage of this document is not allowed unless with written permission from the publisher. All rights reserved.

The information provided herein is stated to be truthful and consistent, in that any liability, in terms of inattention or otherwise, by any usage or abuse of any policies, processes, or directions contained within is the solitary and utter responsibility of the recipient reader. Under no circumstances will any legal responsibility or blame be held against the publisher for any reparation, damages, or monetary loss due to the information herein, either directly or indirectly.

Respective authors own all copyrights not held by the publisher.

Legal Notice:

This book is copyright protected. This is only for personal use. You cannot amend, distribute, sell, use, quote or paraphrase any part or the content within this book without the consent of the author or copyright owner. Legal action will be pursued if this is breached.

Disclaimer Notice:

Please note the information contained within this document is for educational and entertainment purposes only. Every attempt has been made to provide accurate, up to date and reliable complete information. No warranties of any kind are expressed or implied. Readers acknowledge that the author is not engaging in the rendering of legal, financial, medical or professional advice.

By reading this document, the reader agrees that under no circumstances are we responsible for any losses, direct or indirect, which are incurred as a result of the use of information contained within this document, including, but not limited to, —errors, omissions, or inaccuracies.

Table of Contents

Introduction

I want to thank you and congratulate you for purchasing the book, *Hypothyroidism: The Ultimate Guide to Increased Energy, Lasting Weight Loss and Living Well with Hypothyroidism.*

This book contains proven steps and strategies on how to live well in the face of a chronic condition called hypothyroidism so you can gain more energy, lose the hard-to-get-rid-of excess weight, and live fully.

This book will not only provide ways to cope with a thyroid illness but provide significant health teachings. It gives tips on how to care for the physical body and understand the mind-body connection to achieving wellness. The book is written by someone who suffers from this disease and who has lived with it for many years. Once you understand how to live with hypothyroidism, it isn't as complex as you might imagine and is controllable.

After each factual chapter comes a personal chapter to explain what the implications of the preceding chapter mean to you as a patient. I found that when I wanted more information, information of this type was scarce. Of course, there are medical websites, but no one that suffered the disease was talking about it and that's what I needed. Thus, this is my gift to you because I know how much it means to someone suffering. Doctors listen but they don't always hear past the symptoms. Patients, on the other hand, have to live day in and day out with the disease and it can make a great difference to be able to compare notes and know that what you are going through is to be expected, as well as finding ways beyond feeling ill. That's what this book provides.

Thanks again for buying this book. I hope you enjoy it and that you find the information contained in the book a valuable resource to help you to cope with a common disease which is chronic and which affects your wellbeing as well as your health.

Chapter 1:
Background

The thyroid is a small, butterfly-shaped gland front part of the neck. It produces the hormones thyroxine (T4) and triiodothyronine (T3), which acts to stimulate essential processes in all parts of the body. These hormones are extremely important components necessary for an individual to grow, to utilize energy and oxygen, and to generate body heat. They are also necessary for fertility, for immune control in the colon, and for the appropriate use of proteins, vitamins, fats, carbohydrates, electrolytes, and of course water. T3 and T4 can also affect the activities of other hormones and drugs in the body. Thus, you can see that as if affects a lot of actions by the body, it is also likely to make the patient feel quite ill if the balance is not correct. There are two extremes. Hyperthyroidism is when the thyroid is over-active and that can cause hypertension. However Hypothyroid tends to be much more prevalent and can be treated with a drug called thyroxine which is taken regularly at the same time every day.

What is hypothyroidism and when does it occur?

Hypothyroidism is the abnormally low activity of the thyroid gland. This causes growth and mental development problems in children as well as in adults. Hypothyroidism occurs when levels of the T4 hormone go down so low that bodily processes start to become sluggish. This condition was initially diagnosed during the latter part of the 19th century when physicians observed that when the thyroid gland was surgically removed, it led to the swelling of the face, hands, feet, and the tissues surrounding the eyes. This set of symptoms was referred to as myxedema. Doctors appropriately assumed it was the result of the loss of thyroid hormones. More common in people as they get older, hypothyroidism is likely to make a patient feel very sluggish indeed.

Prevalence

There are more or less 27 million individuals in the United States who are found to be afflicted with mild to severe hypothyroidism. A lot more people have not been diagnosed, are misdiagnosed, or have not received proper treatment. Some who were found to have the condition came to realize why it has been disappointing and difficult for them to lose weight. Apparently, this is a severe condition with significant complications for a person in terms of weight and health. Hypothyroidism can affect any age bracket but is mostly found to occur among females who are sixty years of age or older. Medical practitioners observed that most of the time, people who have low functioning of the thyroid are devoid of symptoms like feeling cold or fatigued. These individuals may not realize they have hypothyroidism simply because of inadequate nutrition.

Diagnosis

Hypothyroidism is known to be irreversible and progressive. However, treatment is generally successful which can help the individual experience a normal life.

The condition may either come with observable symptoms or it may be asymptomatic. Diagnosis is found based on thyrotropin (TSH) clinical blood tests. The normal concentration of TSH ranges from 0.45-4.5 mU/L, which is the range for a normal, unaffected person. However, when TSH levels are between 4.5-10 mU/L, the patient becomes diagnosed with mild subclinical thyroid, an indication for early stage hypothyroidism. In this case, despite blood tests that show normal levels, the increased levels of TSH may be attributed to the early drop of T4 levels in the gland. Patients with mild hypothyroidism may or may not experience some fatigue, which is actually very common and affects approximately ten million people in the U.S.

For people with TSH levels above 10 mU/L, they are diagnosed with overt hypothyroidism and must be given appropriate medications for treatment.

Factors that may bring about a higher probability of someone getting overt or clinical hypothyroidism include:

- Being an elderly female, since up to 20 percent of women above sixty years of age are diagnosed with early hypothyroidism

- Having an enlarged thyroid gland or goiter

- Having thyroid antibodies

- Bearing immune factors that indicate an autoimmune condition

It is heartening to note that not all early stage hypothyroidism necessarily lead to overt hypothyroidism. On an annual basis, only about 2-5 percent of people with mild condition develop overt hypothyroidism. Unfortunately, management of this chronic disease has not been conclusive, so steps to cope with this condition must be made known to the general public.

Personal note:

How would you feel is you had hypothyroidism? Well, on a personal note, I experienced a lot of tiredness and I noticed that I was sensitive to heat. I assumed that the heat thing was associated with early menopause. I noticed that I couldn't lose weight easily, though I always had in the past. When summer came, I was usually capable of slimming down for swimwear. However, with hypothyroidism, I was unable to reach goals, which I thought were easy in previous years.

Hypothyroidism may make you feel sluggish. It's very likely to also make you feel like you are less well humored and unable to take things as casually as you normally do. I found that the shortness of temper was something that was strange, as I had never displayed this before and that the lethargy that I felt was very difficult for me to live with. The reason for this is that I had always been dynamic and suddenly I was placed in a situation where I couldn't display that dynamism any more. That hurt and made me feel very old indeed. If you do have any of these symptoms then it's worthwhile getting your blood test. It's a very simple and basic one and the results show the doctor the exact level of your thyroid readings and shows the doctor whether you need to be on medication. When I started, the doctor started me on a low dose that was adjusted gradually. The problem with this kind of medication is that doctors can't afford to make mistakes. If you take too much and your thyroid is pushed too far the other way, it's actually dangerous for your heart.

Another thing that I considered when I was diagnosed were natural things that could help the thyroid and one of these was kelp. Don't do this off your own back. If you can see a doctor who specializes in natural treatments, you may find that kelp will help your thyroid and you will be able to take less medication and that's always a good thing. Your body isn't made for all these additional meds, but in the case of thyroid conditions, you can't afford to fool around. Only use kelp under the supervision of a doctor, because some kelp preparations do little or nothing to correct what you have wrong with you and may be made with such a weak solution that they are really just health food supplies not intended to treat a thyroid condition, whereas a specialist will be able to tell you the right quantities, just like my doctor did.

Chapter 2:
Thyroid Hormones

There are four critical thyroid hormones that regulate how the thyroid gland works in the body:

1. Thyroxine (T4) is the major hormone of the thyroid. When the levels are low, hypothyroidism occurs. On the other hand, increased levels cause hyperthyroidism. T4 is then converted to triiodothyronine.

2. Triiodothyronine (T3) is active biologically but only 20 percent of it is produced in the gland. The other T3 hormones are produced by the conversion of T4 in tissues surrounding the thyroid like those in the kidneys and the liver. When T3 and T4 circulate, they usually bind with proteins that function to transport thyroid hormones. When this occurs, they become dormant.

3. Thyrotropin or thyroid-stimulating hormone (TSH) is released through the pituitary gland. TSH causes iodine trapping and induces production of thyroid hormones. Even at slightly low levels, the pituitary gland acts to secrete thyrotropin to produce thyroxine (T4). Hence, as T4 levels decline, TSH levels go up.

4. Thyrotropin-releasing hormone (TRH) is generated in the brain's hypothalamus which acts to regulate levels of thyrotropin.

Personal note:

When your thyroid hormones are out of synch, all kinds of things can happen. You can feel a swelling in the throat area. I had this feeling and was given an examination to determine whether I was developing a goiter. This is a growth in the neck area. In my case, the tests proved negative. It's not a hard test to go through as it is done by ultrasound and you may find a slight waiting list because there are literally 10 million patients suffering from this complaint to one extent or another within the US, so there may be the need to wait a short while. However, if a nodule is found, your doctor will discuss the treatment he is likely to suggest in your case and refer you to a specialist.

When you see that thyroid dysfunction involves so many hormones, it's little wonder that people's symptoms vary. In my case, I knew that my irritability was uncommon. The tiredness that I felt was also uncommon. Look for symptoms that stand out from the norm because these are clues that there may be something wrong. If you suspect a thyroid condition, you are likely to be suffering from the following symptoms:

- Irritability – in my case quite strongly and out of character

- Tiredness – again out of character, but very present.

Apparently the tiredness occurs because the thyroid condition changes the metabolism, which in turn can make you very tired.

Weakness – this really falls in with tiredness but it's also a kind of lethargy.

Muscle cramps – don't blame this totally on thyroid problems. It may be because you don't drink sufficient water. It may also be that you need magnesium and when my doctor added magnesium to my medical regime and I drank more water, this was less noticeable.

Hair loss or change of hair's condition – In this case, I noticed when I brushed my hair that I was losing more than usual. However, it wasn't to any noticeable extent to outsiders. The one thing that was noticeable was the condition and the need for more conditioner. If you find this to be the case, you can use a coconut oil conditioner to get back your shine until the treatment takes effect.

Memory loss – I put most of this down to age. However, a certain amount of memory loss seems normal though I noticed gaps in my thoughts that were not normal. I mentioned this to my doctor together with all the other symptoms and he could see clearly that there was something wrong and suggested the thyroid test.

If your doctor does not suggest a test for thyroid levels, suggest it yourself because one thing I found was that I recognize within my own body when something isn't right and the blood test was all I needed to be put on the right medication so it's worth it. If the results are negative, you haven't lost anything. You have merely eliminated a potential cause.

Chapter 3:
Insulin Resistance and Hypothyroidism

Some people appear to have a lower need for carbohydrates while some basically consume too much carbohydrate. Some people believe that a low-fat diet means consuming more pasta, bagels, and sweet fat-free foodstuff. Unfortunately, the majority of these items have increased levels of carbohydrates that cause glucose in the blood. Consuming too much of these food items can also bring about insulin resistance and weight problems.

Insulin resistance occurs when the cells turn out to be non-responsive to insulin. Hence, production of additional insulin is needed to maintain the normal levels of sugar in the body. Hyperinsulinemia develops when insulin levels become highly concentrated in the blood.

Resistance to insulin or increased levels of insulin stimulates a person's appetite, making the person crave even more carbohydrates and sugar. This is a quick and sure way to gain weight, and hypothyroidism will make it more difficult to lose the excess pounds since hypothyroidism prevents the body from utilizing stored fat to be used as energy. High insulin lowers the sugar being burned as energy, which makes the cells more prone to store fat and be poor at getting rid of it. It is interesting to note that about 25 percent of normal-weight people and 75 percent of overweight individuals are resistant to insulin.

As mentioned, hypothyroidism slows down the processes in the body up to the cellular level including the breakdown of carbohydrates and absorption of blood sugar. Therefore, when the amount of carbohydrates people consume have become too much for the body's system to handle, this can lead to thyroid problems. For instance, when an individual takes in excessive amounts of carbohydrate, the insulin reacts by causing the body to increase weight. This makes it difficult to lose weight. Moreover, these fluctuations of the blood sugar result to fatigue, lightheadedness, sleepiness, and hunger pangs, among others.

Simply put, too much carbohydrate is tantamount to increased levels of insulin, which corresponds to gaining weight.

Having thyroid conditions and other ailments cause physiologic stress to the patient. This in turn increases the levels of cortisol, and high cortisol tends to increase levels of insulin as well. It then becomes highly likely for the person with mild hypothyroidism to end up developing insulin resistance.

Another negative cycle associated with this is when the thyroid and adrenal glands stop working efficiently, or when the liver becomes ineffective, the body's homeostatic state becomes affected. The liver acts as a go-between among the functions of the pancreas that release insulin and the adrenal and thyroid glands which send signals to the liver to release glucose. The resulting end for all these inefficiencies is increased levels of insulin. When the adrenals demonstrate to be stronger than the pancreas, this can result to the development of diabetes. On the other hand, if the pancreas shows to be stronger, the person may experience fatigue, lowered body temperature, and decreased levels of sugar or hypoglycemia.

This chapter has presented that all the different factors mentioned indicate that insulin resistance is more likely the major causative factor for obese individuals with mild to overt hypothyroidism, as compared to the general population.

Personal note:

In my case, I did have a sweet tooth, and always had. The problem was when I tried to diet. Normally, I could diet easily and bring my weight down. However, you need to change your way of thinking when you have a hypothyroid condition. You don't process food in the same way as you did before. Thus, it's hard to lose the body fat. I found myself changing my diet and making sure that much of what I ate was delicious but that what I ate was in smaller quantities spread out over the day.

What worried me was the fat build up around the waist area and just below the chest. This area was problematic because it meant that I was short of breath for longer than normal. I also found changes to my body temperature and could not tolerate heat as much as I had done in the past. I seemed to get dehydrated easily and had to up the amount of water I drank and also keep medication in the house to activate my electrolytes if they refused to work.

This is particularly relevant to patients who live in warm climates but don't worry too much about the electrolytes treatment. It's made for babies and is obtainable over the counter and really has nothing harmful in it. It's used for sick children to get their electrolytes working again when they suffer dehydration. The quantities that you use are the same as are used for babies and it does get you back to feeling normal again quite quickly. The first time that it happened, I was very frightened because I couldn't bring my temperature down inside. Normally people sweat but it was hot weather and I could not sweat. The treatment brought this back to normal and I make sure now that in summer, it's part of my first aid kit.

Lightheadedness comes and goes and it's different for everyone. In my particular case, I found that it happened quite a lot. By washing my face and freshening up my skin, I was able to make myself feel a lot more human. Another thing that I did to stop me from feeling sick – although this isn't typically a symptom of hypothyroidism – was to make sure that I always had peppermint cordial in the house. This seemed to calm the body down and made me feel a little more normal. I got to a stage where I recognized the lightheadedness and was able to drink the drink in time so that I didn't suffer too much.

The body goes through all kinds of things at the same time because the thyroid affects so many different body functions. Try to cut out as much sugar as you can and cut down on carbs. Try not to replace sugar with sweeteners because these give you a short sugar rush which is false and when you come down again from that sugar rush, you feel even more tired and need more. Thus you end up with too much sugar or sugar replacement in your body. It's counter-productive.

There are a lot of symptoms that you are likely to suffer that the handbook doesn't tell you about. I remember going to my doctor and asking about all kinds of things, but putting two and two together, over the years, I realize now that all these symptoms were caused by the diet that I ate together with the fact that I was hypothyroid. You tend to put a lot of it down to age and make excuses to eat things you like and this doesn't help at all because the fat that's already in your body doesn't shift that easily.

I found that I could do a 16 hour fast to keep my weight in check, and the easiest hours of all were between 8 at night and

14

lunchtime the next day, drinking only water during those hours. This intermittent fasting didn't interfere with my pill taking as I took the thyroxine every day at the same time. However, it allowed my body more time for the daily repair that everyone needs to keep themselves fit and active. It also helped me to burn some of the body fat in conjunction with gentle exercise for the areas that were affected.

Chapter 4:
Steps for Losing Weight with Hypothyroidism

The methods for managing weight of patients with hypothyroidism are not so different from unaffected persons. However, there are some tips to help attain the best overall outcomes:

1. **Be certain that you are correctly diagnosed with hypothyroidism and are given treatment by a professional medical practitioner.**

Obtaining a correct diagnosis and management from a licensed practitioner is vital in the restoration of health and weight management. Diagnosis is based on the laboratory results of a blood test that indicate the level of hormones in circulation. These are T3 and T4 including thyroid-stimulating hormone (TSH). More TSH must be released when hormone levels are dropping. When these hormones are low and TSH hormones are increased, these are indications for hypothyroidism. The exact cut off in reference to the amount of hormones, which determine the condition, is ardently argued.

Recently, is has been proposed by the American Thyroid Association (ATA) that 2.5 mlU/L or higher of TSH indicates hypothyroidism. Other medical physicians base it on a lower cut off point. Most of them still comply with the previous guidelines and look for above 4.5 or 5.5 mlU/L. Physicians usually recommend levothyroxine or synthetic T4 in required doses to restore the body to normal level. More doctors would rather recommend natural medications that contain T3 and T4.

A recent synthetic mix was introduced in the market. The synthetic T3 hormone can be taken by itself or with T4. Unfortunately, T3 is usually overlooked by lot of doctors. In case they do not discuss T3 levels, the patient has the right to inquire because there are individuals who cannot convert T4 to generate activated T3. When T3 is insufficient, it can be very hard to lose weight.

2. Never take thyroid hormones without proper medical consultation

If a patient wants to take these hormones, he should do it with the guidance of a certified physician because there are food items and nutrients that can disrupt how the body absorbs substances. For instance, taking iron or calcium can impede absorption of thyroid hormones. Doctors typically advise to take the synthetic hormone upon waking up or four hours after taking iron or calcium rich foods and supplements.

Also, stay away from goitrogenic foods. These contain components that may impede the functioning of the thyroid. The enzyme peroxidise may be blocked from combining iodine with tyrosine to generate thyroid hormones. Typical goitrogenic foods include legumes, non-fermented soy foods, and raw vegetables like cauliflower, broccoli, cabbage, and Brussels sprouts. When these items are cooked or fermented like the soy, the goitrogen content is reduced. Consuming sea veggies or eating iodine-containing foods can almost always counterbalance goitrogen content in these foods.

3. Have balanced meals with good quality protein particularly during the first important meal in the morning

Having balanced meals with regulated calories daily can help a person with hypothyroidism lose excess weight. All the meals need to include healthy protein amounts. Protein is very filling and as research findings show, it can control hunger pangs more than fats and carbohydrates. It also facilitates preservation of muscles that boost metabolism. The recommended protein amount for a person for the entire day is 0.8 grams per kilogram of body weight.

Breakfast is the most vital period to concentrate on consuming protein since majority of people do not consume adequate nourishment in the morning. This is the period the muscles require the most amount of protein except the hours following exercise. Furthermore, protein sources do not provide similar outcomes for satiety.

4. Consume high-fiber foods, stay away from refined sugars and carbohydrates

Refined carbohydrates only provide empty calories that do not help you lose weight. They do not contain fiber, which is vital for digestion and absorption. Having adequate amounts of fiber is helpful in averting constipation that comes with hypothyroidism. Fiber facilitates satiety, which also helps in diminishing calories necessary for losing weight. The recommended dose of dietary fiber is 25 to 30 grams daily. People who are not used to ingesting these amounts of dietary fiber can increase consumption gradually to prevent gassiness and bloating.

5. Individuals who are resistant to insulin should consume low fat foods and low carbohydrates, with the right amounts of protein.

This indicates that apart from the typical restricted amounts in low fat diet, it is also important to lessen starches and sugars like pastas, potatoes, rice, and bread made of white flour. Consumption of peas, corn, cereal, sweets, dairy, meats, and sweet fruits should also be reduced. This may sound all too disappointing. Nonetheless, it will be very beneficial to curb one's diet towards ingesting turkey, fish, chicken, vegetables with less or no starch, some grains, and legumes. As soon as people who are resistant to insulin begin eating this way, they will start to realize it is not so bad because their hunger for carbohydrates will noticeably dissipate.

6. Exercise daily with resistance training workouts

Engaging in physical activities or lengthy exercise is perhaps the most effective treatment for people who are resistant to insulin. According to research findings, low intensity, extended exercise routines like those that can take an hour will considerably lower levels of insulin. Actually, exercising for a few minutes may be adequate to increase metabolism and use up more calories. These can be done twice or thrice in a day whenever the person's schedule allows it.

Daily consumption of quality protein combined with progressive resistance training can facilitate development of muscles. This will increase one's basal metabolic rate, which means that ultimately the body can burn more calories. Fat takes up more space than muscles, so building them up and losing the fat can make the body fit and lean. A few minutes of exercise a few times during the whole day can also help the digestive process and avoid constipation.

It is vital to remain consistent and not be hindered by hypothyroidism. It is also essential that people are made aware of this fact. They should continue to maintain their health and have persistent goals to achieve their desired weight. If people with this condition have the proper outlook, an appropriate treatment by a medical practitioner, and are also keen on complying with required lifestyle modifications, they can eventually attain well being and overcome this illness. While patients should remain consistent with eating the right kinds of foods and exercising regularly, it is also important to set personal goals and do everything to attain them.

Chapter 5:
Solutions for Increased Energy Levels

Fatigue and experiencing low energy for extended periods are the typical symptoms of a thyroid condition. While hyperthyroidism is typically connected with hyped up energy, it can also cause exhaustion related to sleeplessness, which is a symptom of a thyroid condition. For a lot of patients, an apparent sign that the levels of thyroid are increasing and medications may require changes is the initial indicator, severe fatigue.

In the case of patients with hypothyroidism, even as the levels are within normal range following treatment, fatigue persists. If a person is experiencing waning energy, it is imperative that he takes enough B vitamins. Herbal remedies may be recommended by some practitioners. There are different ways to address the slowing down of metabolism, which can cause fatigue or make the person feel tired. These are the following:

- Do not skip breakfast, which is the most essential meal of the day. If you do not eat breakfast, your body may slow down its metabolic processes.

- Try not to ingest food late at night. Make certain to have light dinners only.

- Avoid starving yourself. Make sure the calories you take do not go under a thousand calories per day. If you do, the body may slow down its metabolic processes.

- Have small frequent meals to maintain blood glucose levels, which result to stable levels of energy.

- Take supplements like Vitamin B12 and other B vitamins.

- Natural supplements are also beneficial like green tea extracts, L-Carnitine, NADH, among others to increase energy.

- Drink enough water to help in the metabolic processes of the body.

- Engage in regular exercises to raise metabolic rate.

- Resistance training twice or thrice a week facilitates muscle build up and increases metabolic rate.

- Avoid goitrogenic foodstuff. Cooking, steaming, and fermenting them can decrease goitrogen content.

- Choose whole foods. They have more nutrients.

Increasing the metabolic rate also boosts energy, facilitates fast healing or recovery, and protects the body from ailments. Other advantages include improving the body system at the cellular level and replacing old cells faster. In fact, new cells may be produced faster at the same time when immune functions improve.

Personal note:

I found that even under these recommendations and with a good amount of exercise, I was constipated, even though I was eating all the right kinds of food. I agree with the findings of professionals about the amount of protein. If you opt for the diet that I am using which is intermittent fasting, breakfast doesn't matter that much as long as you make sure you drink lots of water and eat a good balanced diet with plenty of protein. The protein part is vital. I eat cold chicken, fish, cheese and anything else that is labeled with protein and try to vary my diet.

Since suffering from hypothyroidism the weight loss part is hard work, but it is doable. For example, if you decide to go with what the experts say and have breakfast, don't snack between meals. These snacks may turn out to be your undoing. They were certainly mine. They caused bloating which was excessive and I was constantly constipated.

One diet that I did try for a while which was useful was Special K, because it gave me a whole load more fiber and it was advertised on TV that if you gave up one meal a day and replaced it with Special K, you could lose weight. I am not much of a person for counting calories and find it tedious after a short while, but the Special K diet helped in other ways. It increased my likelihood of avoiding constipation and it helped me to lose a little weight and may work for you. However, if eventually you find yourself bloating, avoid the Special K for a little while because your body may be objecting to too much fiber. You can always do it again once your body has settled down.

Something that you really need to avoid when you have hypothyroidism and something the doctors don't really mention that much is eating too late at night and getting constipated on a regular basis. I started to use laxatives a little too much and found that my bowels were getting lazy and that's not a good sign. If you do find that you are constipated on a regular basis, it's a better idea to change your diet so that it includes natural laxatives such as rhubarb, figs and prunes and if that's not enough, a gentle dose of liquid paraffin from the pharmacy eases your bowels back into action.

I can't stress this enough because the constipation will make you feel overweight because it can last for as much as a week and that's not healthy at all. When you are dieting and you have a hypothyroid condition, it doesn't work the same as it does with healthy people. You cannot rely solely on a change of diet. You also have to change your lifestyle.   That means including regular exercise. If you are a little ashamed of your body shape, like I was, why not try skipping at home with a jump rope, which is good fun and exercises your heart as well, or even try Zumba which is energetic dancing and freestyle. I use a video on YouTube and follow the actions of the dancers on the screen. It doesn't matter if I am no good at dancing. It's the movement and the use of calories that matters and that keeps your body able to keep up with whatever you eat.

It's going to be a hard struggle losing weight when you are hypothyroid, but something you do need to do is make sure that your doctor gives you regular blood tests every two months or so because you need for thyroxine may differ and you may need a higher dosage. They have upped my dosage five times now and I now take 150 µg per day and seem to have been steady in weight for the past six months, which is good news.

If you find your energy levels dropping, get another blood test to make sure your level of thyroxine is correct. If you find yourself having palpitations after your doctor has raised your levels of thyroxine, ask him to re-appraise. I found a very unsympathetic doctor who was standing in for my doctor during a holiday upped my medication by a huge 75 µg in one hit and thought that was rather excessive. If this happens to you, question it because that's a huge increase. The doctor may be correct, but it's certainly worth double checking and having another blood test about two weeks into the change of treatment or earlier if you feel that you are being adversely affected. I knew something was wrong and got mine tested straight away because you should never mess with the dosage of thyroxine since it affects so many body functions.

Chapter 6:
Diet Preferences

There are essential things to consider in choosing food items and beverages when you are diagnosed with hypothyroidism. Remember that your food interacts with medications and the body's general health.

- Soy – This is a goitrogen and it acts to impede absorption of the thyroid hormone. Processed soy and one that has increased levels of phytoestrogen such as supplements, soy milk, shakes, and other forms should be avoided by patients with hypothyroidism. It is critical to only consume fermented soy and in limited amounts.

- Coffee – This beverage is not allowed until one hour after taking a thyroid hormone replacement drug. Coffee can interfere with the absorption of the drug and make the treatment ineffective. The physician may choose another medication that is not affected by this beverage.

- Goitrogenic foods – They contain goitrogens, which can cause goiter or the enlargement of the thyroid gland. These kinds of foods include cruciferous vegetables and soy foods, which can also delay the functions of the thyroid or hypothyroidism. People who are considered to have early hypothyroidism should stay away from eating too much uncooked goitrogenic foods but not necessarily entirely avoid them. They should be cooked first before eating and in moderate mounts.

- Coconut oil – This may be beneficial for hypothyroid patients but it is not an absolute cure. It can be used as substitute for fats and oils.

- Orange juice with calcium – It is ill advised to take this fortified beverage with a thyroid medication. Physicians recommend consuming this juice including iron and calcium supplements only after three to four hours of taking the thyroid medicine. These can impede the absorption of the thyroid drug if consumed immediately after medication.

- Foods rich in fiber – Patients with thyroid condition may also have other issues like constipation and weight gain. They can increase their intake of fiber by choosing high-fiber foods that hypothyroidism patients are allowed to consume.

- Iodized salt – This may be a way to prevent iodine deficiency among pregnant mothers. This deficiency can lead to ailments like cretinism. In the United States, many have veered away from using salt or iodized salt to prevent the increase of sodium levels in the body. This led to a fourth of the entire population to be deficient in iodine. Iodine is necessary for the thyroid to properly function, but it should be used moderately.

- Celiac disease, wheat, and gluten – Celiac disease or intolerance to wheat and gluten may cause autoimmune thyroid condition. When celiac disease patients avoid wheat and gluten, it lessens their bloating and help to increase energy as well as lose weight. However, patients should keep in mind that if they chose to have a high-fiber diet, it is important to have their thyroid evaluated within 8 to 12 weeks. This is to determine if an adjustment of their medication may be necessary because fiber can affect the absorption of drugs.

- Small, frequent meals – This can be effective for thyroid patients in managing their insulin and leptin levels. A lot of people have been made aware that small frequent meals increase metabolic rate. However, this may not apply to patients with thyroid problem attempting to lose weight.

- Drink adequate amounts of water – Among the most effective things people with thyroid condition can do to manage their metabolism and overall health is by drinking adequate amounts of water. This helps improve the body's metabolism, the digestive processes, it curbs appetite, diminishes bloating and edema, and prevents constipation.

Personal note:

Doctors don't give you any indication that food will affect your hormone levels or affect you when you have hypothyroid. Various doctors have treated me over the course of the past ten years and none ever mentioned the fact that coffee affects the efficiency of the drug. There are also other considerations to take into account. For example, Soy products have been linked to breast cancer. Intolerances to foods usually show up much earlier than developing thyroid conditions and fiber may be essential if you are diagnosed as having hypothyroidism because of the constipation factor.

Try to make your food varied. At times you will crave green vegetables and there's nothing wrong with feeding that craving!

Chapter 7:
Live Well Even with Hypothyroidism

The good news is that you can live well even with hypothyroidism. There are lots of therapies available that may be safely integrated with your current treatment. Therefore, patients ought to consider having an optimistic outlook despite their disease. They should choose appropriate foods at all times and empower themselves to live productively. Overall, success is derived from one's strong belief that he or she can overcome this condition. It is a fact that thyroid problems are difficult to completely cure. But it is only up to the person and not the doctors to successfully recover from this health problem. To fully live well, patients can do the following:

1. Determine the appropriate thyroid treatment.

You may be one of the patients who are suffering from hypothyroidism and examining which treatment is more effective to you among levothyroxine, T4T3 therapy, or natural methods. It is imperative to determine the appropriate treatment. For some patients, anti-thyroid medications are unable to alleviate hypothyroidism symptoms and they cause certain side effects. Nowadays, surgical procedure is becoming a better option.

Knowing the right medication and right dosage is not an immediate process. This may need some trial and error procedures; hence, it is necessary to develop patience. It is possible that some people who were diagnosed with hypothyroidism tried different brand names of the drug levothyroxine, integrated synthetic T3, and considered natural supplements. With trial and error processes that may be performed periodically, it may be easier to find the right therapies for the individual. This may be wearisome but once the right treatment is found, it will be worth it.

Personal Note: It took a very long time to find the right medication and even though it was found, from time to time this needs changing because the thyroid condition changes. The only way to ensure that you are making the right choices and have the best possibility of living happily with the condition is to ensure that you have a doctor that cares enough to test you regularly so that the levels are kept under control. The synthetic T3 isn't something that is immediately offered to all patients. I had to fight to get it and did find that it was able to help me to some extent control my weight better than without it. I still think that it's only a matter of time before surgical treatment will follow though for the time being have the illness pretty stabilized. If your doctor doesn't give you regular blood work, then you may need to insist on it. Some doctors are less sympathetic than others and do not seem to realize the changes that this illness is making to you. Therefore, it really is up to the patient to ensure that they are being treated correctly.

2. Choose the right physician.

It is important that the patient is confident with his or her physician. It is an important part of deciding to live well. If you are currently being treated by a bad practitioner, do not hesitate to divest yourself of this person. However, there are situations that you are dependently stuck with the only option available. You may have to deal with an HMO physician or with the only specialist residing within your locality. If you can do something about it, try your best to locate a good physician who can actually help you and be your willing partner as you work toward wellness.

Personal note: In this situation, I found myself with perhaps three different doctors who didn't take the condition that seriously. One didn't offer blood tests unless I insisted. Another upped the dosage sufficiently to actually threaten my life and another was so lethargic in her treatment that I decided my life was worth more than that. You have to decide on the following criteria:

- Is the doctor giving you regular checkups?

- Does your doctor adjust your medication if necessary?

- Does your doctor offer alternate medicine if you need it?

Do you have a doctor that doesn't think you are being neurotic? The last one is particularly relevant. Sometimes, when you have hypothyroidism, you may seem a little fussy but it is the illness that is making you feel that way and a good doctor should understand that. Look out for a doctor that does because this is a real treasure and will make all the difference to your treatment. If you get one that simply thinks that you are neurotic, expect to go through the mill with different treatments even before they suggest testing you for Hypothyroidism. Insist on it because you need a doctor that is interested enough to make sure that your medication is always at the right level and that means regular blood tests.

3. Understand your thyroid condition.

You can be empowered by educating yourself. This is also important so it becomes easier to have a grasp of what your physician is trying to tell you during consultation. You have to take responsibility in understanding what your body is going through by asking relevant questions, talking about options with your health care provider, and looking for another physician if the current one seems ineffective. Researches and studies about this condition are continuous and so medical discoveries may crop up anytime soon. If physicians are getting this kind of information, you also have the right to be informed especially if recent discoveries are about your thyroid problem. There are also numerous resources online and offline.

Personal note: If you do seek information online, don't believe everything that you read and don't suddenly start to associate symptoms with what you are reading. If the symptoms are really there that's one thing, but reading Internet websites about your illness can lead you to developing symptoms that aren't really there. The danger with this is that your doctor does not then know your true condition. You can even believe all the symptoms that you find are due to thyroid problems but you may be wrong. I remember finding one symptom on a website and believing that it was due to the thyroid, but I was wrong. It was caused by another illness altogether, so don't try to live your illness. It is controllable and the medications hide most of the symptoms.

The responsibility you should take is asking to see your blood work tests and keep a record of them. These show the evolution of your illness and if you do get to the stage where surgery is considered, all of this paperwork is very useful to the surgeon. If you forget to take your medication, don't double up on the next dosage. Simply write it off to experience and make sure that from tomorrow onward, you do take the correct dosage at the right time and without using coffee as the drink of choice to take it with. Remember, you are cutting down the efficiency of the drug if you insist on taking it in this manner.

When you understand your thyroid condition better, it's not so scary any more. At first, I wondered what to expect but the most spectacular change you are likely to see is lethargy if you need your medications adjusted upward and palpitations if it needs adjusting downward. It's actually not that usual to adjust in a downward direction and is more common that as you get older, you need more thyroxine treatment rather than less. When you are aware of the way that you feel and have a label for it, it's actually not that difficult to live with. Yes, I get sluggish times when I am very tired, but I always know what the cause is and it's usually brought about by forgetting to take my daily thyroxine tablet.

4. Help others learn as well about this condition.

Part of living well despite having a thyroid illness is to help others become well informed also. Other patients may have erroneous beliefs about this ailment. Not too many individuals understand this condition. All they probably believe is that this disease makes older women overweight. This is a biased and imprecise description that may cause for some physicians to misdiagnose patients. Make certain that like you, other patients and significant others understand the disease. In a way, you will be doing your part in raising awareness.

You can begin by educating the members of your household and the community you belong to. Members of the family of patients diagnosed with hypothyroidism also need to be informed so they can offer more patience and understanding to their loved ones who have the condition. They can also help their family member to comply with the right lifestyle modifications required to improve health and wellbeing. Sometimes you will be coming across people who do not understand the disease or may have erroneous beliefs about it. You should take the time to clarify things to them, which can be very helpful to other patients whose family members lack the knowledge and understanding.

Personal note; One of the reasons for writing this book is so that people can see from my own vast experience of the disease that it is livable with, but that you need to be vigilant. This is your life and you have a responsibility to yourself to ensure that you look after your body in the best way possible. Thyroid problems are a pain when you first have them, but after a while they become part of who you are and just change a little as time goes by. As long as you are aware of those potential changes and make people around you aware, that's what's the most important. In fact, friends have asked me about the illness because we are all different and sometimes as a hypothyroid patient, you feel a little isolated with the illness because, as stated above, people take for granted it's a woman's problem that makes her fat. It's much more than that.

By explaining to people that you know about what the illness entails, you raise awareness and help them to deal with family members who also have the same problem and may not yet have discovered how to live with it. My sister, for example, seemed to develop this quite young and wondered what on earth was going wrong with her health. A very energetic person, she suddenly found herself lacking in energy and pretty lethargic about life and was almost treated for depression. When I mentioned that it sounded like hypothyroidism, her attitude was strange because she didn't believe she was old enough to suffer from it. However, she called to thank me when she had been diagnosed and treated because she suddenly felt like her life was back on track again.

By the way, did you know that hypothyroidism is genetic? It can be passed down through the family so don't forget to talk

34

to family members about it. However, not everyone within a family will get it. Out of a family of 6 kids, only three of us have it. It's quite likely to be more than one kid in the family that will develop it. Thyroid problems come from a lack of iodine in the body and there's not much you can do to correct that.

5. Remain steadfast and determined to overcome the thyroid condition.

As a patient, it is imperative to remain steadfast in the face of illness, difficulties, and hardship. Although there are great therapies or medications, total cure does not happen overnight. Hence, patience is necessary during all the phases of treatment. However, patience does not mean that patients should be passive. Among the most difficult facets of a chronic illness like hypothyroidism is the necessity to be serene and at the same time determined. It may be easy to give up, but it is wiser to keep on trying to look for the right solutions, right physician, and the right mode of treatment.

Personal note: Since you have a thyroid condition because of lack of iodine, it would be reasonable to suppose that iodine supplements should help you. However, be aware and never self-medicate. I once did this was very ill as a result. That's one of the downfalls of reading up on your own illness and thinking you have the expertise to translate what you read on the Internet and in books.

If your doctor believes that introducing iodine may help you stem the effects of hypothyroidism, they are likely to introduce this in small measure by the use of kelp tablets. I mentioned these earlier because my doctor believes in the use of plants and natural elements. However, she also knows that it's necessary to start the dosage in small quantities because you can't mess with something like the thyroid. The other thing is that you will be asked by a caring doctor to undergo a urine test to check whether it's working but it only works in conjunction with the other missing factor when you have hypothyroidism and that's selenium. Don't second guess your doctor because you are playing with danger.

The thyroid touches so many different functions of your body and it's vital that you don't self-medicate. Even if you are short of money, try to ensure that you treat your hypothyroidism in a responsible way through a caring physician, rather than trying over the counter meds that may even make you worse. I say this because experimenting yourself is likely to make you feel worse.

Your body is reacting because of the lack of iodine but you don't know how much and it's dangerous to assume that introducing iodine will help as you don't know the how your body will react and absorb any iodine taken. Don't just assume you can experiment blindly and simply taking a selenium tablet at the same time may not work because unless you are expert on doses, it's better not to mess around with your health. Let a caring doctor oversee any changes in the medication that you are taking.

6. **Make sure you have personal support from family and friends.**

Part of living well with this health problem or any chronic ailment is to obtain support from those who are willing to offer this and be there no matter what. These people can be the members of your family, friends, colleagues, and support group affiliates. They can all take part in supporting and egging you on to be healthier and capable of managing your illness. People who do not believe you have an ailment are not helping. This may happen at work when your boss does not provide support to the fact that you are not in good health and may need proper medical attention and time for treatment.

The most effective support providers are persons who do their best to gain knowledge about your thyroid condition, so they are able to be patient and understand your needs. Sometimes it is necessary to encourage people close to you to accompany you for consultation so they can ask questions and be aware of what is happening to you while suffering from this condition. This can make challenging periods easier to understand.

There are numerous support groups online and offline. Be wary and make certain you do not partake in groups that exclusively concentrate on symptoms without considering the solutions. There are groups out there that only intend to sell medical products or perhaps have biases or opposing views on talking about all available options. Some groups do not consider natural or complementary alternatives for treatment. So make sure to make adequate research about the groups you plan to join in.

Personal note:

If, like me, you start to find yourself irritable and snappy, warn your family that it's your illness that is making you like that and to expect changes once the medication has been adjusted. The irritability seemed to hit me at different times of the year and I was never sure why. However, I didn't accept that I was merely getting older and more miserable. I knew that something was amiss.

Explain to your family members so that they are more understanding of your illness. You never know, they may have inherited the illness and may demonstrate it later in their lives so the better the understanding of it, the more capable they will be of seeking the right kind of advice when it happens to them. I found that talking about it was particularly useful because it meant that they had a better understanding of what was happening to me. Many people go undiagnosed but you give your loved ones more information by being open about the illness. When and if it happens to them, they will recognize the symptoms and are much more likely to get themselves a caring physician to deal with the illness rather than merely ignoring it and leaving it untreated.

My family was my support and yours should be too because these are the most likely people to notice changes. For instance, if you are particularly bad at taking your meds, get them to give you a daily reminder. Don't let your prescription run out as this treatment is almost always for life. I have been told by my doctor to expect to take the treatment permanently and something that I always do is check any new medications against thyroxine to make sure that it's suitable to be taken when you are diagnosed as having a hypothyroid condition.

7. Avoid taking daily stresses too seriously.

Stress is one factual occurrence in life that can cause major impact on one's chronic condition like hypothyroidism. It can worsen the person's illness and may change the body's requirement for thyroid hormone. Hence, dosage adjustments may be necessary because the fixed dosage is no longer adequate. When a person is stressed, the brain produces substances that can cause depression, anxiousness, and other health problems. If stress is diminished, there are changes in the body's immune system and brain that can improve the body's capacity to overcome illness.

Personal note:

I find that this description of hypothyroidism is very accurate. You can take the stresses of life too seriously and I found that when I did, I was getting very light-headed and wondered to myself whether I was nearing a stroke. It was that apparent that it gave me concerns. However, at times when stress was less noticeable, I was able to calm down. What I ended up doing was leaving a job that was stressing me because it made me so ill and that helped a lot. However, I have also had many adjustments to the medication. Do not assume that all of your symptoms are from hypothyroidism because you can develop other disorders as well.

Just go to your usual doctor and explain what's happening to you. When you do manage to go relatively stress free, you actually begin to feel normal and if you are in a high stress position, I would suggest for your own benefit that you try and cut down those stresses to actually feel reasonably healthy, rather than weathering them out and going through a very bad patch with your illness. It's really up to you to handle it but it scared me when I was lightheaded and it was my own fault for allowing the stress to build up to such an extent.

When I learned to lower the stress levels and not subject myself to this kind of stress as well as having hypothyroidism, I found that life became a lot easier. If you are someone who stresses, the things that can make a difference are things like joining a yoga class where you are taught how to balance body and mind and are thus less likely to expose yourself to undue stress. Meditation did me good but on other fronts as well. I became more confident and actually found that I was able to make decisions about my career with a much clearer mind because of the meditation practice.

If you do feel lightheaded, I have a tip or two that can save you going through all that worry. Lightheadedness feels frightening because you wonder if you are having a stroke or something like that. Keep yourself hydrated particularly in hot weather. Don't expose yourself to too much stress from walking in the heat of the afternoon sun. I found that really did bring on the lightheadedness. If you do suffer from lightheadedness, the best thing you can do for yourself is simply lie down in a quiet place and practice your breathing in through the nose, hold the breath, and then out through the nose at a peaceful rate which helps you to get your blood pressure steady.

The thing is that lightheadedness can seem scary and when you are scared, your blood pressure level goes up. The more you worry about that feeling – and it can be pretty scary sometimes – the higher your level of blood pressure until you find yourself in full panic mode. You need to switch off that process and simply lie down and breathe because you soon get back to the condition you should be in. This happened to me several times and the first time, I even called out an ambulance. From the blood test taken at the hospital it was clear the hypothyroidism had been the cause as there was no other cause pinpointed during extensive tests.

The second time that it happened, I was aware of how I was making the situation worse by being worried about it. If you do feel this way, lie down in a cool room and just breathe. It does pass and more quickly if you adapt a sensible approach and don't get yourself into a state of panic about what's happening to your body.

8. Have an optimistic attitude and view on things.

More often than not, having an optimistic emotional state is extremely helpful in fighting off the disease condition and even lengthen the patient's life. This report came from a scientific research study. The idea is that the more positive the outlook of a person is, the less stress is placed on the body. If stress is diminished or reduced, the body is able to thrive successfully, is enabled to fight off any infectivity, and is able to obtain more resources to dedicate to healing and recovery.

Personal note: I don't take life that seriously these days. I know I am getting older and accept that deterioration is part of that process. I laugh about it because there's not much you can do to stem it, but I do know that when I compare my attitude toward life and my sister's, my attitude is healthier. She tends to live her illness and uses it at any possible time to explain why she behaves in a certain way. Personally, I think if she dropped the thought of living the illness, she may actually free herself from feeling so bad much of the time, but she is younger than me and will learn with time what best suits her body. I am an optimist. I am not the kind of person to take pills at the flip of a hat because I have headache or because my leg hurts. I tend to be very wary about introducing anything to my body that it doesn't actually need. By being able to drop stress and have a generally healthy outlook on life, it is easier for me to live with hypothyroidism. The only time I blame it for anything is when I find I can't lose weight in the summer, but my partner is also getting overweight and out of shape with age, without having hypothyroidism, so I suppose we all have that cross to bear.

If you can keep upbeat, you don't let your illness take over. It's strange, because much of the time my body tells me what it wants in the way of food, rest, exercise, etc. and I have learned that by listening to it, I don't suffer that much at all. When your body does send you messages, and you have hypothyroidism, it pays to listen. I think one of the ways in which I got in touch with my inner self was when I started to meditate. This meditation helped me to relax but it also made me a much stronger person and that helps with a disease such as this. It makes you more aware of your body and tells you when something isn't quite right. Whenever I have voluntarily gone to the doctor and asked for a blood test, I have been spot on with being aware of changes in the thyroid levels and an adjustment fixed the problem.

One thing I will always be a little angry about is the lack of seriousness that some doctors have when treating the condition. For example, no one told me that you can't take thyroxine tablets with coffee and for years, I was swallowing them with my morning coffee at breakfast and that accounted for the fact that they didn't make me feel that much better. They should be taken with water and at a distance from drinking coffee. There are many medications that have their power reduced by coffee so if you are a coffee head like me, try to make sure that you take your meds separately and that you don't use your coffee with which to swallow them. Simple explanation by a sympathetic doctor may have made the first two years of living with the disease a lot easier.

9. Aspire to really live well.

On the whole, to live well with hypothyroidism means making a firm decision that you will become the person who goes through life with optimism. It is important to feel confident that someday you will successfully overcome this condition. Ultimately, the person may learn to live with this problem and at the same time lead a healthier lifestyle. It is imperative to work around the disease or its debilitating consequences, or possibly even reverse the condition and completely treat it. But in the course of this journey, you have to choose to live well. It is necessary to be practical and at the same time realistic. Some health problems do not have an absolute cure, but that should not impede you to continually seek for healing. Never get worn out or frustrated, and never quit.

You are the only person who gets to decide if you have really done all the things you can possibly do and want to do to improve your health and how you feel. You are the only person who can say you have dedicated enough of your time, consulted the best physicians you can reach, tried almost all medications recommended, used different diet regimens, sorted out the mind and body connections of chronic illness, and others. Having tried everything in your capacity, the step that should follow is for you to accept your situation, and then move beyond that kind of limitation. You can now decide that it is high time to concentrate on getting healed, rather than being cured. You can allow yourself to let go and move on. You should not be hindering your own progress. And while moving on, be accepting of the fact that there are others who have offered support to you during your distress and are still continuing to be right by your side as you continue your journey.

Certainly, there will always be good times and bad times in seeking health for individuals with hypothyroidism. However, one facet that cannot be changed by any treatment or physician is your own will to live your life to the fullest. Even if one's health may have control over a person's way of living and the other way around, it is you who possesses the strength to live well.

Personal note:

I think that one of the best things that you can learn when you have hypothyroidism is to check your neck on a regular basis and if you feel that you may be developing nodules, ask for an examination. I have only thought that twice in 17 years so it's not a big deal. However, it's always possible that you will develop nodules and that these may have to be surgically removed. One friend had the operation and is as right as rain now and said that it was the easiest surgery she ever had and that she was out and about very soon after the surgery. Personally, I haven't had it and perhaps will never need it.

I found one thing since being diagnosed that helped me and that was changing my diet. I used to eat a lot of things that were fattening and perhaps merited a little of my overweight problem but find that as long as I am reasonable with my diet and don't overdo it on the sweet stuff, I can still have the odd treat and get away with it. I am fortunate in a way because I was never overly big anyway. My sister, who has large breasts, finds it harder than I do because she always looks bigger so if you are large breasted, you may need to take more care with the food that you eat. I found that trying all different kinds of tastes, I actually enjoyed some things that were very healthy and made me feel good, so do experiment with food. There is other food out there than sweet food even if you have a sweet tooth.

Do try your doctor for the integrated synthetic T3 if you find that you are putting on an unacceptable amount of weight. Doctors may not volunteer it and may just be accustomed to dishing out Levothyroxine, which is a standard medication for hypothyroidism. However, if you have a heart condition, be aware that the T3 can actually make your heart beat faster and perhaps your doctor was being prudent in not prescribing the drug. However, if you cannot lose weight and you find the symptoms of hypothyroidism are too much to live with you could discuss with your doctor the use of the slow release variety and make sure that you always take it with a full glass of water so that it is dispersed in the correct manner. You need to take some precautions with your diet if you are concerned about putting on weight because of hypothyroidism and the next chapter is devoted to ideas that don't mean too much sacrifice on your part but that can make a difference. You also need to incorporate exercise into your life and there are some suggested exercises that may help you to beat the extra weight.

You have to live with the disease once you have it but it doesn't have to make you into a cripple. It's not crippling unless you decide to overplay your illness and it is very manageable. The bit you may not like is not being able to lose that weight as fast as you would have done in the past. However, this only began to affect me when I reached over the age of 60 and was living a much less active life. As previously stated, this book is my way of helping those who have discovered this illness and if you have been diagnosed and are in your early years, remember that as you get older it gets harder to lose weight. Thus being prudent with your diet is important now, not in the future – when things get too hard.

Chapter 8:
Substitute Foods and Exercise that will help

I think it is very important as soon as you know you have a hypothyroid condition that you prepare for what is to come. Although you may have a sensible diet and take a reasonable amount of exercise, in view of the dangers of gaining weight, it's a good job to actually prepare so that at an older age, you don't find that you are in danger of getting diseases such as diabetes. The problem with the thyroid is that it acts in so many parts of what your body does that if you continue to eat sweet things and starches on a regular basis, you can make your own situation worse. I wish that someone had told me that back when I was 40. It would have made life a lot easier in the long run, but they didn't.

Try to learn about substitutions of food that will help you in other ways as well. For example, swap butter for Omega 3 type spreads, cut out red meat as much as possible. Cut down on the type of milk that you use and low fat milk these days is much more palatable than it used to be. Change coffee for decaffeinated coffee because it makes you less excitable. It's also a good idea to eat a variety of vegetables and fruit to keep your body working like it should. The problem is that you can get very constipated with hypothyroidism and it can become habit forming. It is far better to use natural methods to ensure that you are regular and eating the right kind of fruits will help you.

Try to substitute white bread for whole grain bread because once you get accustomed to the taste, you are actually giving your body a lot more goodness. I found that eating fish on a regular basis also helped considerably as this is brain food but it does more than that. It is filled with Omega 3, which is exceptionally good because it stops you from developing high cholesterol levels. My doctor also swears by the fact that an apple a day keeps cholesterol levels low. If, like me, you have little tolerance for peeling and eating apples, try buying freshly stewed apples in a jar because these are just as good.

As far as how much you eat is concerned, cut down your portions because the only inevitable thing about hypothyroidism is that you will gain weight and it won't be in the places you want to gain it. Skinny people generally do not suffer from hypothyroidism and if you ask others who have the same condition, you will find that the percentage of people who gain weight because of hypothyroidism is exceptionally high. Thus, if you take precautions from the moment that you are diagnosed, you can actually make a difference to the outcome and not have to go to drastic measures to lose those extra inches. The places that I found I put weight on the most were in the waist area and stomach.

To counter the effect of this, I downloaded an app for exercises, which are used to get rid of the belly area, and they were very successful indeed. I also did Zumba, which helps all the parts of the body and expends a lot of calories but I wasn't a slim person and would have been embarrassed to do this with others. I therefore opted to do it alone at home. This got all my energy levels up and eventually persuaded me to join a yoga club. A yoga club is a great addition to your social life as well because people seeking to balance out the way that they feel use yoga practice to help them to achieve this. I am not much good at advanced exercises, and that's being honest with you. I do, however, get an awful lot from the meditation exercises and the sun salute and find that these put me in a very positive frame of mind.

Since doing all of this, my mood is enhanced. My energy levels are also higher and although I am not my ideal shape yet, I seem to have stemmed the weight gain. For a while, during working in an office, I decided to treat myself to salads that were already prepared and could be bought in supermarkets and found that light lunches, as opposed to succumbing to temptation of bagels and suchlike did me the world of good. I didn't feel heavy in the afternoons and found that I was much less prone to changes in my thyroid levels that necessitated a change of medication levels. That to me was good news.

If you need support and help locally, it's a good idea to ask your doctor if there are support groups as these can help you by showing you that you are not alone. I didn't need a support group because I had a great family to back me, but if you find that you are living on your own then these are a good idea because you share ideas and also get to know others with your illness that can give you great advice. I visited one group for one particular evening to give a talk on hypothyroidism and people were very grateful for the talk because until that moment, they had thought that all of their symptoms were actually neurosis rather than being anything to do with the thyroid. As doctors downplay the effects of the thyroid, you do need to be aware of what the thyroid can do to you that you may not be expecting:

- Yes, you will gain weight

- Your hormones may mean that you get emotionally upset more frequently

- You may even feel depressed

- You can feel hungry at strange times. Try to curb nighttime eating.

- You may feed too tired to exercise. This is a battle you have to go through

- You may feel that people don't understand your illness

- You may feel isolated and alone

- You may feel lightheaded and wonder if it's something more serious

The point of telling you this is that if you decide to take yoga lessons, it's a good idea to let your yoga teacher know that you suffer from hypothyroidism. You may be wondering why but there are exercises that are especially aimed at improving your thyroid levels which you can see on lowthyroiddiet.com, but which you shouldn't really try alone. The best thing about these is that there are videos and if you ask your yoga teacher to go through these exercises with you, you may find that you can improve your thyroid readings just by doing these exercises on a regular basis.

This is particularly relevant to those who have been diagnosed young. Don't give up on your body and don't wait until you have gained so much weight you don't have the energy to exercise. Since these exercises are designed particularly for people with hypothyroidism, they are the ideal exercises to help you in your newly diagnosed condition and an instructor can show you how to do the exercises in the correct way, helping you with posture.

I found that posture had a lot to do with how I felt and it's a time to stop slouching. If you constantly slouch, the places where you will gain the most weight will really be noticeable, as your tummy will look bigger than it actually is. Learn to sit straight and keep your spine straight. This is the right position for the breathing exercises your yoga teacher may want you to do but it's also ideal to keep your figure in trim for as long as you can.

If you mull over the pages of this book again, you will be able to use it to guide you through your illness. I have covered everything that I can think of from the medical practitioner point of view and then from my own point of view as a patient. I have also based observations on other patients who suffer the same illness so chances are that somewhere in this book you will find answers that will help you to live with your hypothyroidism in an easier way than I did. In the next chapter, we relate to some resources for people who have discovered that they have hypothyroidism and these will be useful in particular cases as listed.

Chapter 9:
Top Thyroid Resources

After years of research and a quest to find the top thyroid health experts, I am in the best health ever. I spent countless hours online searching for the most valuable information. Here are links to top resources that every person with hypothyroidism (and every person who suspects they have it) should check out.

1. If you're pregnant and have hypothyroidism, you should have your levels tested every four weeks. However, this doesn't apply to those who are not pregnant. If the links are in a printed book, just copy them into your browser for more help. This resource is useful for people to gain a better understanding of thyroid problems.

   - http://www.everydayhealth.com/thyroid-pictures/hypothyroidism-causes.aspx#/slide-4

2. **Thyroid Pharmacist**

   - **http://www.thyroidpharmacist.com/**

This website has a lot of up to date news on thyroid conditions and may be useful for people who want to know more about their illness than this book has given. With a blog and supplements, the site can give you good value when you are looking for solutions.

3   **Reflexology**

   - http://media-cache-ak0.pinimg.com/originals/3f/26/b7/3f26b74bd1d9d8b86b8121efb091f405.jpg

Ever thought about reflexology? This could be a solution to your problems. The link above shows you how.

4. The Five Most Harmful Thyroid Myths

- http://thyroid.about.com/od/gettestedanddiagnosed/a /The-Five-Most-Harmful-Thyroid-Myths.htm

Just as you learn a lot of information online, you can also learn things that worry you. Put a stop to all the myths by reading this document that can help you set aside the myths so that what you are learning is the facts.

5. Adrenal Fatigue Related Health Conditions

- http://www.drlam.com/blog/adrenal-fatigue-related-health-conditions-part-1/2854/

This resource may be interesting to those who suffer from fatigue and who want to find out which health conditions may be responsible for that lack of energy. It's quite likely to be hypothyroidism if you have already been diagnosed but there are other illnesses so checking can be a prudent thing to do.

6. The connection between Fibromyalgia and Hypothyroidism

- http://healthimpactnews.com/2011/the-connection-between-fibromyalgia-and-hypothyroidism/

This may also make interesting reading. Many people who the medical world cannot label in any other way are now told that they are suffering from fibromyalgia. In fact, what this means is non-specific arthritis or arthritis that doesn't have any other name. It's worth finding out if your aches and pains are related to your thyroid condition, but remember that you can up the energy levels and get rid of a lot of aches and pains by drinking regular water and by taking up yoga with an instructor who is conversant with the yoga exercises specifically targeting those with hypothyroidism.

7. **Hypothyroidism and the Role of Armor Thyroid, Seaweed, Exercise, and More -- Cutting-Edge Interview with Joseph Mercola, D.O. / Thyroid Disease Information Source - Articles/FAQs**

- http://www.thyroid-info.com/articles/mercola.htm

8. **Practitioners Share Their Approaches to Optimal Hypothyroidism Treatment**

- http://thyroid.about.com/od/hypothyroidismhashimotos/tp/Top-Doctors-Share-Best-Ways-Treat-Underactive-Thyroid-Hypothyroidism.htm

This is a link that takes you to medical resources shared by professionals and it may answer some of your questions on your condition.

9. **Dr. Alan Christianson - Weight loss for people with thyroid disease**

- http://drchristianson.com/blog/

10. **Baywatch Star and Thyroid Patient Advocate Gena Lee Nolin has a great following on Facebook and Twitter. She is a person to follow.**

- http://thyroid.about.com/od/publicawarenessoutreach/a/Baywatch-Star-Thyroid-Patient-Advocate-Gena-Lee-Nolin.htm

Conclusion

Thank you again for purchasing this book!

I hope this book was able to help you realize your goals in helping yourself and others have more patience and understanding of people with a chronic thyroid condition. The way that I have tackled the situation is by showing you the medical view and the patient view so that you can see that you are not alone in your struggle against all the effects of hypothyroidism. At times it will seem like an uphill battle. At times you don't feel anything but normal and at other times, the fact that your hormones are all out of balance can really play havoc with your logic and make you feel even more ill than you should. By making yourself more aware of this in advance, you stop that from happening because you take control. When you do that, you put yourself in charge of your body, even though your body is defective and is giving you problems.

You can do that. It's very similar to taking precautions when you have a bad leg. You rest it or give yourself a crutch. In the case of hypothyroidism, you just need to rest when you need it and fight off the fatigue that will eventually lead to weight gain. If you can do that, there's no need for the illness to be at all crippling. Although your doctor may have described your condition as "chronic" many people misunderstand that word. All that means is that your illness is ongoing. It doesn't mean it has to restrict your life or that you need to worry about it. All you do need to do is be aware of the potential of weight gain, fatigue and perhaps even depression and try to keep yourself motivated, knowing it's the thyroid's problem rather than something you have to deal with.

The key takeaway is that now you armed with more information regarding thyroid health. This book covered a number of topics including:

- Thyroid Hormones

- Insulin Resistance

- Steps to Losing Weight

- Increased Energy Levels

- Diet

- Living Well

- Top Thyroid Resources

But in each chapter it also included personal comment which was thyroid illness from the patient perspective using many years of experience as my guide to help you see things the way that patients do and thus gain a better understanding of your ailment.

My suggestion is to go back and read parts of the book that most spoke to you. Take notes; do further research if necessary but most importantly, begin applying these ideas into your life. When you do that remember that the feelings I have experienced may not have happened to you and if you are fortunate may never happen to you. The most common elements that you will share with me with your hypothyroidism are going to be weight gain and tiredness.

There are many tips within the book to help you overcome these problems because they can become large problems that are difficult to deal with if you let them get out of hand. If you change your usual pattern of behavior to adjust for your new illness, however, life can carry on and it can be very challenging and exciting. Hypothyroidism is not the end of the world. It's a condition that you can treat with meds and that you can control by your choices of actions to take to contra the negative effects. If you do this even before they happen, you may never have to go through these effects and will be able to live much more easily with your hypothyroidism than I was.

The purpose of this book was to give you a resource I didn't have. Yes, there were the odd forums where people complained about their bodies a lot, but the point with these was that the patients involved in the discussions did very little to help their fellow sufferers. Sometimes these places can be hives of negativity, which is not what you need when you have a newly diagnosed condition.

One such forum had me believing that it was almost automatic that hypothyroid patients will become diabetics and that is of course nonsense. That's why I thought that putting together constructive advice based on medical fact and patient experience was far more helpful to those seeking information. This is my way of saying thank you to the doctors who have helped me to deal with this illness and to the people like my yoga instructor who have helped make this illness have much less significance.

Preview of "Thyroid Diet: A Natural Thyroid Diet Solution Plan to Restoring Your Health in 30 Days or Less"

This entire book can be downloaded by clicking on the following link: http://amzn.to/1acqrtx

Chapter 5:
The Natural Diet Solution Plan for Better Health in 30 Days (Or Even Less!)

The main component of the Solution Plan described in this book is hinged on the nutritional component of the health restoration process. All medical practitioners have a vocal consensus on the importance of nutrition on the overall health and well-being. The diet plan in Chapter 5 is, therefore, effective either for those who have hypothyroidism or those who have healthy thyroids and would like to go on a preventive intervention against thyroid imbalance.

Nevertheless, bodily processes are complex. When one party is afflicted with disease, the smartest approach towards recovery is to consider all possible avenues for intervention starting with the naturals. Natural healing usually does not entail use of pharmaceutical medicines that are either invasive or non-invasive treatment types. Instead, a healthy diet and positive eating habits plus physical activity and lifestyle modification are encouraged to restore and maintain health. This is the Solution Plan advocated in the book.

The following scientific facts were considered in the formulation of the natural Solution Plan for thyroid problems:

- Stress is a contributing factor in the over-secretion of the hormone cortisol. Cortisol is the body's natural anti-stress formula. When an individual is stressed, the body produces more cortisol. The problem with cortisol is that it blocks many of the thyroid functions. This usually results in thyroid imbalance.

- In addition to cortisol, its precursor called corticotrophin-releasing hormone (CRH) also tends to inhibit the production of the thyroid stimulating hormone (TSH).

- Cortisol also hinders the conversion of the inactive thyroid hormone T4 to the active form T3. A reduced level of T3 can cause hypothyroidism.

The first phase of the Solution Plan, the 30-day thyroid diet, has been presented in Chapters 3 and 4. The remaining phases of the plan are discussed in this chapter as recommendations.

Engage in Medically-Supervised Regular Physical Activity

It is, of course, understood that exercise is a challenge for thyroid patients because of the fatigue factor. Impairment of the thyroid functions takes its toll on the body's strength and vitality. Working out is an issue. Those who have developed goiter already have trouble breathing.

Never embark on a physical activity program unless you are cleared by your doctor. Usually, doctors can give you a referral for a fitness specialist, particularly an exercise physiologist that specializes on people with thyroid problems. Since there are various disorders that lead to thyroid problems, the exercise routine for thyroid patients should be customized for their unique case.

Walking is always one of the best exercises. Walking will not pose any danger to thyroid patients as long as they do not overdo their routine. It is, however, more reassuring for both the thyroid patient and his/her family if this is OK with the doctor and how much time will be safe.

Taking Care of the Adrenal Glands

Avoid overworking your body. When people attempt to take in more workload than they can handle, they tend to get stressed. Excessive stress overworks and overloads the adrenals and causes them to weaken.

Never derive energy from inappropriate sources. Caffeine and sugar also takes its toll on the adrenals. Refined foods also deplete the body of B vitamins, which is necessary to have healthy adrenals. If you want energy and vitality, eat healthy and engage in physical activity. Always start your day with a good breakfast and a healthy disposition.

To maintain healthy adrenal glands, avoid the following foods:

- Caffeine;

- Chocolate;

- Cola;

- Refined foods such as: bread, biscuits, burgers, cakes pies, and pizza;

- Sugar;

- Tea;

The following are adrenal-friendly foods:

- Fresh fruits and vegetables except the restrictions that have been outlined in Chapter 2;

- Licorice;

- Quality proteins, except fish. Consult with medical and nutritional professionals regarding the inclusion of fish in your diet;

- Vitamin E-rich foods such as avocadoes and wheat germ;

- Whole grains (Reminder: control your servings)

Embark on Lifestyle Modification

If you confess to have lived a hazardously stressful life, you can restore your good health with a fairly reasonable lifestyle modification. This is a case-to-case basis. The stressors that affect you are not necessarily the same stressors that affect other people. However, it is the position of this book that running away or coping with your stressors does not work anymore for more people. You need to face your stressors with a new weapon – a lifestyle and behavior modification.

Work is always the main stressor for most people. Nevertheless, avoiding work is no way to relieve stress. Otherwise, you will be dealing with additional stress because of boredom or financial difficulties. You have to realize that work is just an element of your stressor. It is not work, but too much work. You do not need to run away from work. You just need to know when to stop stacking work in your office desk, say no to sideline projects, and say no to weekend overtime. You are human; you need rest.

Maintain your Health

The analogy of maintaining your health can be made to a follow-up consultation with your physician. You would have observed that your specialist makes it standard practice to schedule you for a follow-up visit even if your present check-up indicates that you are already well from your illness. The doctor might also prescribe maintenance medication to ensure that you are completely healed of your illness.

In all probability, as long as your thyroid problem is one which doesn't need surgery or radiotherapy, or simply put, as long as your thyroid problem is detected early and has not caused serious complication, the Diet Plan and Solution Plan that comes with this book will help restore your normal thyroid function in the course of 30 days or even less.

Celebrate! However, never miss out on the maintenance plan.

Chapter 6 concludes the Natural Diet and Solution Plan for your thyroid problem with the final phase which is Maintenance.

The rest of this book can be downloaded by clicking on the following link:

http://amzn.to/1acqrtx

Check Out My Other Books

Below you'll find some of my other popular books that are available on Amazon and Kindle as well. Simply click on the link below to check them out.

Thyroid Diet: A Natural Thyroid Solution Plan to Restoring Your Health in 30 Days or Less

- http://www.amazon.com/Thyroid-Diet-Solution-Restoring-Influenced-ebook/dp/B00EOAV6QY

Dash Diet Action Plan and Recipes for Busy People: Lose Weight, Lower Blood Pressure and Feel Amazing!

- http://www.amazon.com/Dash-Diet-Action-Recipes-People-ebook/dp/B00G07D694

Paleo Lunch Box: Quick and Easy Mid-Day Paleo Diet Recipes for Health and Wellness

- http://www.amazon.com/Paleo-Lunch-Box-Influenced-Practical-ebook/dp/B00ENPWUME

Paleo Breakfast Recipes for Busy People: Quick & Easy Recipes to Help You Lose Weight, Feel Healthy and Look Amazing!

- http://www.amazon.com/Paleo-Breakfast-Recipes-Busy-People-ebook/dp/B00F3NC49O

New to Paleo: A Beginner's Guide to Super-Charged Health with the Paleo Diet

- http://www.amazon.com/New-Paleo-Beginners-Super-Charged-Breakfast-ebook/dp/B00DE6FN9K/

Bonus Offer for Free Books

If you're interested in receiving updates on new books and free book promotions, please click the link below:

https://docs.google.com/forms/d/1ttDqtdRjOeAEtA-BKnq5Hw668vjQSoVWcXCGQ8z9frA/viewform

One Last Thing

When you turn this last page, Amazon gives you a chance to rate this book. If the book was able to help you to find solutions, do tell others because they may, just like you, be looking for a good resource to give them information about their illness. Your few words of review could make the world of difference to other patients. Be honest, be kind and remember that you are not alone in your struggle. With so many patients suffering from this chronic disease, you won't be the last either, but by spreading education among family and friends, you can make it a disease that people are able to live with and cope with in a much easier manner.

If it helps anyone in some small way, they'll be forever grateful to you, as will I.

There is always a glut of information on the Internet. Through Amazon, it has become possible for people like me to write sincere books that address the suffering of people from all kinds of illnesses. I am grateful for the books that I have read on cancer in an attempt to help friends who were suffering from it. In fact, one book that I read was written by a sufferer and that gave me the idea that perhaps that's what was needed for hypothyroid sufferers as well. This is my gift to them and I have read through to make sure that I am giving readers the best value they can get, seeing the illness presented in the most comprehensive way possible. Thank you for reading my book and sharing my experiences. I hope that yours are easier to go through in some small measure because of what you read within the pages of this book. Thank you.

Health writers who do suffer from illnesses may be making a stand these days to provide the public with the best information that they can get. If you find that you still have questions once you have read the book, the resources in my chapter devoted to resources are extremely useful ones and the best of the bunch. Enjoy. Even if you are not reading this in your Kindle or mobile device, you can still type the addresses into your browser and find out what's being said currently about the treatment of your illness, thus keeping up to date with developments.

CPSIA information can be obtained
at www.ICGtesting.com
Printed in the USA
LVHW041540090223
738974LV00007B/393